Food Addiction, Binge Eating

And Hypoglycemia

How To Overcome It

And Get Your Body Back To Balance

From a Survivor

How to get your body back to balance, stop cravings, food addiction, fatigue, low energy, depression and mood swings

How to get back the energetic life which is your birth right and gain a healthier, more vital body

First Edition
March 2015
Golden Bay
New Zealand

Tony Clearwater
PO Box 334, Takaka 7142, New Zealand

Legal Disclaimer

To the best of my knowledge, the information contained in this book is accurate

This book is for 'reactive hypoglycemics'. For helping heal hypoglycemic symptoms from sugar addiction and stopping food cravings and mood swings.

Diabetic hypoglycemia is a more specialised subject and isn't fully covered in this book. Diabetic hypoglycemics should talk to their doctor first if they want to follow any advice from this book.

If you take any prescription medication talk to your doctor before doing the 'cleanse' or if you want to stop taking them. There may be withdrawal symptoms

Pregnant mothers should also talk to their doctors about any steps they may follow from this book as they may need additional supplements. They should avoid the 'cleansing diet' or any fasting

Tony Clearwater

Contents

Chapter One

My Story

What Is Hypoglycemia?

Symptoms

6 Quick Steps To Start

1. Stop Eating All Processed Foods

2. Balance Your Blood Sugar Levels

3. Add Enzymes, Vitamins and Minerals

4. Use Proper Food Combinations

5. Exercise

6. Reset Your Emotional Trigger Point

Chapter Two

Hypoglycemia

- How To Get Rid of It

- Why Vegetables, Can Save Your Life

- The Importance of The Liver

- Foods To avoid For Now

- Bread

- Meat

Chapter Three

Use Foods That Heal You

- Make Salads More Interesting

- The 'Super Salad'

- Fruit Salad As A Meal

- A Bit About Fruit

- Alkaline Foods

- Try New Foods and Meal Suggestions

- The Short 'Cleansing Diet'

- Don't Eat Too Late at Night

- Find Your Natural Appetite

- What To Drink?

- Feeling Hungry

Chapter Four

Other Helpful Information and Techniques

- Skin Brushing and the Lymph System

- Take Notice of How You Feel After Eating?

Chapter One

My Story

Binge eating is an addiction. I've never been a heroin addict but I often compare it to this. It's a craving that you can't stop. Remember the Nutty Professor when he reached into his desk drawer for the Mars bar? And the uplifting symphony music that started playing? That's how it is for me. It's like I try to have will power and abstain from sweet foods, but then in one glorious suicidal capitulation I give up. I'm going to die anyway so I might as well enjoy myself - I think we've all been there.

Food addiction is an illness. Many of us have our addictions whether its alcohol, drugs, sex or food. Why are we like that? There are various theories. For me I think I got off to a bad start. I was only breast fed for 2 weeks. So my Immune system may not have been as strong as it could have been. My mother left when I was three, she didn't like my father and my birth was very painful. She took my sister and never let us meet. Telling my sister lies that her Dad didn't love her. I met my sister when I was 26. I went to thirteen different schools, Dad went through another divorce. Any of these things may have affected me in some way.

I was brought up on the usual kiwi fare of weetbix processed cereal, milky puddings and lollies. This is my addictive food - I like sweet milky things. I could drink a whole can of sweetened condensed milk when I was young, and I regularly had peanut slabs, milkshakes and ice creams. I was very physically active so it didn't seem to bother me. Except that I had some emotional problems, which seemed to be made worse by the food I ate.

I would cry a lot, I was anti-social and had black moods and suicidal thoughts. I was depressed and felt sorry for myself. I didn't know it yet but these are all symptoms of hypoglycemia. I was a mess. And even though I had some good jobs like being a raft guide, I still couldn't maintain a balance in my life

I reached a peak when I was 26. I was working full time building and orchard work. I couldn't figure out why when I came home for lunch I would eat a Swiss bread sandwich with cheese and salad, a healthy lunch I thought. But then I would collapse on the bed feeling exhausted. After work I could eat a whole packet of chocolate biscuits and then another. I felt great at the start but afterwards I would feel disappointed with myself and lousy. I had learnt that if I made myself throw up I would then feel a lot better. This went on for a year and a half - and then I found a book.

It was just a short little book on hypoglycemia. I had heard of it but didn't know what it was. The first page had a list of symptoms that went on for the entire page and I had all of them. I felt a little better about myself. I wasn't a complete freak and a loser. I actually had a very common and recognised illness. I managed to heal myself in two months. Buying my first mountain bike helped.

I was at a good point for many years but slowly slipped back into it. I peaked again when I was 42. I was house sitting for some friends for ten days. I found a 2 litre tub of ice cream in their freezer and I decided to eat it and replace it. I didn't have TV or a couch at my housetruck so I lay on their couch watching TV and eating ice cream. I ate and replaced that 2 litre tub of ice cream five times in ten days! My big toe began to swell up and that was the start of psoriatic arthritis which affected my mobility and my life badly for many years.

What is Hypoglycemia?

I don't know if all binge eaters are hypoglycaemic, but I would guess that most of them are. To learn about what it is you need to learn about the pancreas and what it does. The pancreas produces insulin, so when you eat sugar your blood sugar level rises. This is the 'feel good' moment. Your pancreas produces insulin to bring your blood sugar level under control and stabilise it. All well and good, but if you're hypoglycaemic your body is stressed and out of balance. The pancreas becomes overworked and overactive and it produces too much insulin, sending your blood sugar level diving to below where it should be

This is 'reactive hypoglycemia' caused by an overactive pancreas and binge eating. Hypoglycemia can also occur if you are a diabetic and your insulin levels drop too low. Or by 'fasting hypoglycemia' which happens by going without food for too long, drinking alcohol or by too much exercise which lowers the blood sugar levels

- Reactive hypoglycemia is the one which creates a continual cycle of moodiness, cravings and depression

- Fasting hypoglycemia is short term and can be more easily fixed with some carbohydrate and sugar

- Diabetic hypoglycemia is usually caused by taking too much diabetic medication which causes insulin levels to drop too low. Hypoglycemia for a diabetic can lead to seizures and a coma. If the person is conscious eating very small and regular amounts (20gms) of carbohydrate or sugar will usually help until you can see a doctor

This book is for Reactive Hypoglycemics

It's about the common cycle of binge eating and sugar addiction. You get a craving which only sweet food can fill. You gorge yourself on sugary foods and immediately feel great! But then you come crashing down and feel terrible and have low energy.

Of course you may not be addicted to sweet food. Maybe your craving is for savoury food. Roast chickens, pies, bread and butter and pizza. The information in this book will work for you too, though there are a few particular things to help the sugar addicted hypoglycemics.

If you're a savoury binge eater your body is still out of balance and it needs to rest, detoxify, cleanse, stabilise and get back into its natural state

Testing for hypoglycaemia

Your doctor can give you a glucose test to see if you are hypoglycemic. If the test shows you are, you may be showing serious signs such as dizziness and shakiness. But … if the test shows you aren't hypoglycemic you can still be showing the milder, early symptoms. It's possible that you may not be clinically diagnosed as a 'reactive hypoglycemic' but all of the information in this book will still work to balance your body and give it a well needed rest, stopping food cravings and getting full on hypoglycemia later on

Why Are We Out Of Balance?

There are several reasons. One is your addiction which is often caused by an emotional problem. Most addictions are created by us to block out and suppress emotions we don't want to deal with. This is one of the basic premises of Alcoholics Anonymous.

I also need to mention here that some addictions may be caused by prescribed medicines. Complications arising from the side effects from these medicines is something that will most likely be more common in the future. And weaning yourself off painkillers, anti inflammatorys or depression medication may help you. Consult your doctor first and tell him your plans. But for now let's just talk about the common food addiction to suppress emotions

So why are we out of balance? My theory is this:

Mental and Emotional Reasons

- We have a food, or drug addiction to block emotions we don't want to feel
- We may be deeply unhappy, depressed or dissatisfied with our lives, feel like we are a failure or overly compare ourselves to others

Physical Reasons

- Our bodies are overworked , overreacting or sluggish
- Our bodies are over acidic
- Our bodies are craving vitamins, nutrients and minerals
- Our stomachs are overstretched and we've lost our natural appetite
- Side effects from medication

Symptoms of Hypoglycemia

These aren't limited only to hypoglycemia but they can be a good indicator:

Anti-social behaviour, black moods, crying for no reason, fatigue, pale skin, heart palpitations, anxiety, irritability, shakiness, hunger, sweating, dizziness, sensitivity to light and sound, inability to make decisions, stressed

7 Quick Steps To Start

Before I get into details I know you want a quick fix so here are some things you can do right now.

1. Stop eating all processed foods including white bread, pastries, ice cream, lollies and packaged foods loaded with preservatives and additives.

This may be a hard thing to do if you are a heavily addicted savoury binge eater. If that's the case then don't worry, we have a few tricks up our sleeve so that you can still enjoy some of those foods you love.

But you need to get your body back into its natural appetite and balance and this will be very hard to do if you continue over eating on these foods Processed food such as white flour don't provide much fibre and it can make you feel sluggish and 'gum up' your intestines. Your body will be working hard to digest it. The excessive refined carbohydrate of white flour converts quickly into glucose and then glycogen by our liver – and unless you're busy running a marathon this glycogen will be very quickly converted into fat, usually on our thighs, buttocks and abdomen. This is what is called a 'High G.I. food or High Glycemic Index.

White flour, refined sugars and saturated fats are the worst culprits and they make the liver work very hard.

But make sure you eat regularly. This helps maintain our blood sugar levels. You just need to eat food that's good for you. Whole grains with vegetables will provide a steady supply of energy which is less likely to convert to fat or cause mood swings

2. Balance Your Blood sugar Levels

For Sugar Addicted Hypoglycemics

If you think you are hypoglycemic from sugar addiction these foods can particularly help

Foods which naturally balance our blood sugar levels.

The most beneficial of these are natural liquorice twigs. Yes liquorice actually comes from a tree and you can chew on the twigs. I used these and they do get rid of the cravings

Ask at your local health store. If you can't get them there just buy liquorice tea or Red Seal Blackadder tea. It's slightly sweet and if you drink it after a meal or when you feel a craving it will help

Other foods which naturally help balance blood sugar levels are avocado, maple syrup, almonds, Greek yoghurt, green tea, cinnamon, turmeric, cider or white vinegar, kale, spinach and all fibre rich vegetables, apples and citrus, beans and chickpeas, fish, nuts

3. Add Enzymes, Vitamins and Minerals To Your Diet

This one little trick will help start your body back on its road to health

Both Savoury and sweet bingers can start by buying those little packets of dark, small leaved salad greens. Even if you don't like them, don't worry. I will teach you how to like them later. Alfalfa Sprouts can also be used

One of the reasons you are craving food is because you are undernourished. These salad leaves are packed with not only vitamins and minerals but with enzymes. Straight away you can add a few of these leaves to your pizza, meat pie or roast.

If you don't like mixing them with your favourite food, force yourself to eat a handful of them before you begin. This one trick alone can kick start you onto your road to recovery. Those of you who love salads will just have to bear with me for a while as I have to aim this book to the large group who don't like them!

Here's why this trick helps ...

Enzymes

Enzymes are a key to health and nutrition. These magical chemicals are what help us digest food. If we are stuffing our bodies with lifeless, processed foods and white flour, our body has to work hard at producing enough enzymes to digest the food. The more help we can give our body the more energised we will feel and the more nutrition we can get from the food we eat

By eating a small amount of these nutritious green leaves either with or before our meal, our body will be able to digest proteins and starches more easily and it will also obtain the rich vitamins and minerals present in these dark leaves. Even if you don't like them - it's only a few seconds of suffering while you munch them down and then you can enjoy that greasy pizza! But now you should feel better afterwards.

At the end of eating you won't feel as tired and you should feel lighter and more energised

I try to eat a small amount of enzyme and vitamin rich foods with each midday and evening meal. Besides greens there are sprouts and any other vegetable you can think of which can be eaten raw. This is Important because the enzymes are destroyed at 38 degrees from memory, just above body temperature

Of course you can grow your own salad leaves of mesclun lettuce, rocket, mizuna, mustard leaf, sorrel etc. or sprout alfalfa, mung beans, sunflower or almost anything

4. Use Proper Food Combinations

Your stomach requires a different enzyme balance to digest a carbohydrate meal compared to a protein one. Eating salad greens will benefit both

Carbohydrates in particular can be hard to digest as they need to go through three different processes. The first digestive process begins in your mouth with the enzyme ptyalin in your saliva, so chew your food well

Start a little experiment. Try eating either a protein meal such as meat, fish or tofu with vegetables or greens or a carbohydrate meal such as rice, pasta or other grains with just vegetables or salad. You should notice that you feel lighter and more energised afterwards

This is an ideal food combination

- Protein / Vegetable or Carbohydrate / Vegetable
- No proteins and carbohydrates together
- Eat fruits on their own. Don't mix with starch / carbohydrate
- Milk products ideally should be eaten on their own

This is the ideal. So your typical hamburger is not an ideal food combination. But I don't want to get religious about it. The more natural and pure your food is, the better your body will be able to digest it. So it's not too great a crime to add a little tofu to your noodles or small pieces of bacon to your pasta

Dairy products should be eaten on their own, but small amounts can be added to either of these combinations.
Sugar will of course upset the enzyme balance a little, so try to avoid sugar rich foods until at least 20 to 30 minutes after eating or even one hour.

Fruit requires a different enzyme balance and should be eaten separately
Also avoid drinking too much before or during a meal as this will dilute the enzymes

5. Exercise - Take a Walk

Our bodies like movement and this can really help get your body back to its natural balance and importantly - help you find your natural appetite.

Personally, I'm a little lazy – I don't like cycling but I do enjoy walking. Its gentle and I find it peaceful and meditative so it's good for my head. I try to find somewhere close to nature and I will sometimes do an active walk swinging my arms. You can also try swinging your arms from side to side like some Chinese do; this activates your core and internal organs

Yoga is great. It will force feed and pump blood into specific areas of your body, cleansing and revitalising it. I wouldn't recommend doing any postures where your head is upside down though while you are going through this cleaning phase. You may be feeling giddy and your blood could have toxins in it which can cause headaches

Of course any sort of cardiovascular exercise is beneficial – it gets the heart and blood pumping which helps your body get rid of waste and cleanse itself and will often help reduce inflammation. But try not to exercise too hard or for too long as this can lead to low blood sugar levels

As you can see I'm a great fan of walking but any exercise will do. I had a cross country training machine once which was great until I broke it. Exercise which works your core muscles is also very good. But whatever you do, don't overdo it and be gentle on yourself while you heal.

6. Reset Your Emotional Trigger Point

The basic premise is this – When we get a craving its usually caused by an unstoppable wave of emotion combined with a churning sensation and pull in the stomach. This becomes a pattern and a habit which can be very hard to break.

One way to stop it is to trick your body and get it to snap out of this all-consuming feeling. There are various ways and some are simple such as –

- Wash your hands, forearms and face in cool water

- Go for a swim or have a luke warm shower

- Have a bath with epsom salts

- Do any sort of exercise or sing loudly

Hypoglycemia

How to Get Rid Of It and What To Eat

The first thing to do to get rid of hypoglycemia is to stop eating sugar, refined, processed carbohydrates and white flour. These foods overburden your liver with sugar and your overstressed pancreas is going haywire flooding your blood with too much insulin, this in turn sends your blood sugar levels diving and gives you mood swings and more cravings. Use the liquorice twigs or liquorice tea to balance out your blood sugar. If you need some sweetener use a little natural maple syrup or rice / nut / oat milk.

The basic idea is very close to the steps in this book:

- Cut out all pastries, fatty meat, dairy products, sweets and processed food, fried food and junk food, juice and snack bars. Even dried fruit and very sweet fresh fruit

- Eat mostly easy to digest grains such as millet, buckwheat or quinoa, vegetables, salads and healthy protein such as tofu, nuts and fish

- Eat smaller meals more often to maintain your blood sugar

- Carry healthy snacks of slow release carbs or protein such as nuts or wholegrains or bananas

Baked vegetables are okay. Try to avoid frying and steam your food, it's much healthier. Cook your vege's in a covered pan with a little water and near the end lay some fish on top to steam. This is a much healthier way to cook than frying which can create harmful, cancer causing compounds

When adding olive oil or butter to foods, try to do it at the end of the cooking so that the oils don't get damaged

Drink enough water and use liquorice tea or twigs to balance your blood sugar levels

When I kicked my hypoglycemia I would soak ground cashews, almonds, sunflower and sesame seeds overnight and then drink the milk. This was fantastic and it satisfied my craving for sweet milky foods. The remaining pulp could be mixed with sea salt and herbs to make a savoury pate

These days there is a wide variety of almond, oat and rice milks. I use these in moderation. It may not be perfect but its way better than buying a milkshake and it satisfies my sweet tooth

Why vegetables can save your life

Vegetables and fruits are storehouses of vitamins and minerals, and these vitamins and minerals are carried in life's magical and wondrous ingredient – water. The water borne nutrients in these foods make it very easy for our body to absorb them. Our bodies are made mostly of water and the building of cells and removal of waste from our cells also happens through water via osmosis and the lymph system. So it makes sense that our bodies will work well by eating foods with water in them

Personally I can feel it – I just feel good after eating a meal with vegetables. I'm not saying I love vegetables - I could like a good bacon sandwich as much as anyone, but if I'm honest and want to talk about how I feel after eating certain foods - then I feel best after eating a light meal with lots of vegetables or salad. And if you add a few condiments it can taste better than meat

I already let you know about my secret - that I'm lazy. I could live off sandwiches all day, they are quick and tasty. But I end up putting on weight and feeling bloated. So I force myself to cook a decent meal of a whole grain quinoa, rice, pasta or other grain at night with a tasty sauce and lots of veges. Another good meal for my body is steamed fish with broccoli and salad or coleslaw. And if I'm in town I pay $8 for a mixed salad of greens and various whole grains such as beans, chickpeas or potatoes.

The Importance of The Liver

The liver is the largest organ of the body and it filters 1.4 litres of blood a day. It has several important jobs

- Cleanses your blood and gets rid of toxins

- Regulates carbohydrate metabolism

- Regulates protein metabolism

- Turns glucose to glycogen and maintains your blood sugar levels

- Produces bile to digest fat

- It's the only organ in the body that gets rid of fat

Symptoms of a sluggish and poor working liver can be :

High blood pressure, fluid retention, hypoglycemia, inflammation, circles under the eyes, a coated tongue, bad breath, bloating, chronic fatigue syndrome, headaches, migraines, gallstones

Poor liver function can make asthma and hay fever worse. Saturated fats are also hard on the liver and should be eaten sparingly. These include all animal fats, butter, whole milk products, cheese, fried foods, takeaway foods and processed foods. In saying that, there is an argument saying that a small amount of natural saturated fats can be healthier than factory made oils.

Healthy fats for our liver include the omega 3 and omega 6 oils which also have anti-inflammatory properties.

Omega 3 oils are Fish, salmon, herring, tuna, mackerel, shrimp, oysters, soya beans, walnuts, pumpkin seeds and canola oil

Omega 6 Oils are Sesame and sunflower seeds and oil, corn, raw nuts, soya beans and spirulina

Some foods which help detoxify and regenerate the liver are kiwifruit, grapefruit, green tea, garlic, leafy greens, turmeric, avocado, walnuts

Supplements that are very beneficial to the liver are:

Lemon juice in the morning or Swedish Bitters with water will activate the liver to start cleansing itself. If you don't like lemon juice mixed with water, try drinking the lemon juice on its own first. Preferably combined with some light exercise or a brisk walk. The liver is most active between midnight and midday

Psyllium hulls

Slippery Elm Bark – mix 150 to 1000 mg with juice. Slippery Elm is soothing on the intestines and useful for gastritis or stomach ulcers

Dandelion tea or leaves

Carrots and Beetroot, which contain the antioxidant beta-carotene

Foods To Avoid For Now

If you are hypoglycemic your body is stressed and out of balance. Its overworking and your digestive system will be weak. You will most probably feel and look bloated. These are foods which are a little harder to digest or just have too much sugar and it may be good to avoid them for now especially if they make you feel bloated.

Rice and lentils
White rice is a high GI food and will quickly flood your body with sugar which will be stored as fat. Use brown rice in moderation
For a change try baked vegetables such as potatoes and pumpkin. Baking makes them easier to digest. Or Quinoa, millet, polenta or buckwheat

All fruit juice and dried fruit.

The sugar is too concentrated and it will trigger hypoglycemic reactions. It is okay to add a few sultanas to a curry. Use fresh fruit in moderation

White bread, sugar and commercial honey
Local honey is more likely to be unheated and healthier. Use a very small amount in drinks if you have to. Natural maple syrup is better

Sweetened yoghurt - This is just lollies mixed with milk. Try unsweetened Greek yoghurt which is high in protein. Swap full fat cheddar cheese for cottage cheese

Bread

I'd like to make a small mention here about bread. These days there are some wonderful whole grain loaves being made but they are not cheap at around $8 a loaf. For years I ate a Swiss style loaf thinking it was good for me, but this was basically white bread with whole grains mixed with it.
I noticed that these whole grains seemed to come out intact at the other end, and I suspect that they also absorbed water from within my body as I became very constipated. Use in moderation

Meat

Lean meat is the best to use. Fried or barbecued meat is very hard on your liver and any blackened animal meat or fat can be damaging to your body and can contain cancer causing compounds

Now is also a good time to think about the welfare of animals. If you've ever seen them being crowded into a truck and taken to the slaughterhouse it can be hard to watch. Think about the pigs and chickens crowded into sow crates and battery cages, where they are stressed and can hardly move. Do you really want to support this?

I was a regular meat eater and I know how it is. You think meat is the most wonderfully satisfying food on earth and you just couldn't live without it. But after a while I really started to notice the flavour. And I have to admit that I find vegetarian food is far more flavourful.

The country I live in, New Zealand, has one of the highest rates of bowel cancer in the world. And we are the world's third highest meat eaters the last time I read the statistics. It's not uncommon for many kiwis to eat meat three times a day. The people with the lowest incidence of bowel cancer in the world are the nations who eat very little meat and more vegetables.

Animals such as dogs that predominantly eat meat have very short intestines and food stays in there for only five or six hours. Humans have very long intestines which aren't designed for a high meat content diet.

A little lean meat two or three times a week is probably fine as long as its eaten with some vegetables or salad to help it move along. "But our cave man ancestors ate a lot of meat" I hear you say? I'm sure they had times where animals were scarce and they used every edible plant, seed or fruit they could get. And they didn't have the luxury of walking down a supermarket aisle everyday that's laden with every different type of packaged meat. I would imagine that after the first post hunt meat eating frenzy they had to subsist on a lot of healthy vegetables and roots!

Of course it's hard to give up completely if it's been a large part of your diet. And I believe that small, incremental changes are more long lasting than sudden ones. So maybe just cut back on it and explore other alternatives. And if you have a craving, add a small amount to your salad or meal. But think about the animals.

20

Chapter Two

So How Do We Fix It?

Now you've read the Seven Steps above you are off to a great start. You've already learned a little about:

- Enzymes, Vitamins and Minerals
- Why you should cut back on white flour and processed foods
- Proper food combinations
- Eating small but regular meals
- Gentle exercise and cardiovascular exercise
- Changing the emotional 'trigger point' which creates cravings
- Foods which naturally help balance our blood sugar levels

Now let's go into it at more depth and talk about some more techniques ... This may seem daunting. But everything is broken down into easy steps

Basically we are talking about giving your body a chance. Give it a rest from all the processed foods. Give your liver a rest so it can detoxify and rejuvenate itself (this can help stop headaches) and give your pancreas a chance to heal and balance itself

Eating salad greens with good food combinations and reducing our sugar intake will rest our body and help it start to recover, getting it back to its natural balance

Use Foods That Heal You

Make Salads More Interesting

Some of us like salads and some of us don't. For those who struggle with them here are some things you can do. First, get used to the bitter taste of some leaves. If you eat a few at the start of the meal, the common thought is that it will stimulate bile production which will help digest fat. By eating a few greens first we provide a rich enzyme environment to help digest our food

Some Tips

- Add a sprinkling of raw or toasted sesame, sunflower or pumpkin seeds to your salad. Pumpkin seeds are rich in zinc which is essential for the hair, nails and brain

- Add wedges of avocado or tofu or even sliced boiled eggs, tuna and croutons as you would to a nicoise salad

- Grated carrot, beetroot, fresh corn or celery

- A small amount of honey

Experiment with buying different dressings or learn to make your own

A basic simple dressing could be:

Finely chop or squeeze some garlic (optional)
Mash it in a small amount of oil
Add 1 to 1½ half cups of olive or sunflower oil
½ cup of cider, balsamic, white vinegar or lemon juice
A little salt and pepper and/or some herbs

As a last resort, if you're craving something substantial you could add a good quality mayonnaise or grated cheese. It's not ideal but it's one way to ease the adjustment into a more pure, raw food diet.

The 'Super Salad'

As you can see from above, it's entirely possible to use your salad as your main meal in a mostly raw food combination. The super salad is another version of this. The idea is to make a complete meal using more than one form of protein as a base

For the main base ingredients use either organic pre-cooked or cook yourself kidney beans or any other type of beans, chickpeas or lentils.
Add to this some chopped raw veges from your garden such as celery and parsley, grated carrot and beetroot. Add some steamed dark greens and maybe some avocado and sprouts

Now add something to liven it up – some marinated, grilled or baked tofu, grated cheese or eggs. If you're a big meat eater this is a good way to start weaning yourself off meat. Add thin strips of beef, chicken or bacon.

Fruit Salad as a Meal

This can be a little heavy on the stomach. But try mixing chopped apples, bananas and kiwifruit with something tasty like some sliced citrus or grapes. Then mix in some tahini or a few chopped almonds or pine nuts. On top of this can be added any of the following - lemon juice, grated ginger, cinnamon, carob, coconut, pumpkin or sunflower seeds

A Bit about Fruit

As I just said, eating sweet fruit may not be helping your hypoglycemia, but I think it's worth it for a short time to gain the benefits of a full body cleanse. All fruits are helpful but ones I find particularly beneficial are –

Peaches
I don't know why but in season peaches seem particularly good at cleaning out your insides

Kiwifruit
These are one of the best. Get organic and unsprayed if you can. Kiwifruit are rich in enzymes and have been recently proven to be one of the few foods that helps to regenerate liver cells

Grapes
A great intestinal cleanser. If you can't get organic and they are imported, wash them in a little warm water and a small amount of eco-friendly detergent

Watermelon
A gentle but very effective intestinal cleanser. Watermelon is also a diuretic meaning it will activate your kidneys, helping cleanse them and shed your body of excess fluid. Watermelons should be eaten on their own and apart from other meals

Papaya and Pineapple

Not everyone likes Papaya or Pawpaw but I love it. Along with Kiwifruit it is one of the most enzyme rich fruits and its particular enzyme, papain, helps to eat up old protein waste from our bodies. Pawpaw will definitely help you shed some kilos.

Pineapple also contains another powerful enzyme, Bromelain. You will feel it going to work as soon as you eat it but be careful. Pineapple is quite acidic and it can form some painful cracks in the corners of your mouth if you overdo it

On the subject of acidity, most fruits are acidic but they will have an alkaline reaction in your stomach

Apples

Nature's miracle cleaner and weight loss remedy. Try to get organic ones. If you can't then peel the skin and don't eat the seeds as the skin and seeds are where the majority of spray and toxins are stored. The toxins from a sprayed orchard are hard for your body to get rid of and it tends to accumulate them. Apples are good for diabetics

Pears and Plums are great gentle cleaners.

Bananas

You wouldn't think of bananas as cleansing but they have many beneficial properties. They are high in fibre and loaded with potassium which helps to make the body more alkaline. Try them split with peanut butter

Try to get fresh fruit in season. It will be more effective than fruit that may look good but has been stored in a chiller for nine months

Alkaline Foods

The modern day human body has become very acidic from eating processed, refined and junk foods.

What are alkaline foods? Most fruit and vegetables are alkaline. Even acidic fruit will have an alkaline reaction in the stomach. Here are just a few examples:

Alkaline Vege's: Broccoli, cucumber, celery, lettuce, leafy greens, kale, onions

Alkaline Fruit: apple, banana, grapes peaches, melons, berries, lemons, citrus

Alkaline Proteins: almonds and tofu
Alkaline Grains: buckwheat and millet
Alkaline Spices: Cinnamon, Curry, Ginger, Mustard, Sea Salt

Symptoms of an over acidic system:
Teeth that chip easily, pale skin, tiredness, ulcers, acid reflux, cracks in the corners of the lips, dry skin, leg cramps, headaches, tendency to infection, feeling cold, depression

Sea Salt is also slightly alkaline and cider vinegar mixed with water is also beneficial for alkalinising the body

Try New Foods and Meal Suggestions

Now is a good time to learn about new foods and how to cook them.

The alkaline grains - buckwheat and millet can be used in both sweet and savoury dishes. They will help to cleanse your body. There is also a whole array of new, ancient grains which are packed with essential proteins and nutrition such as quinoa and amaranth. Polenta is cheap, tasty and good for both sweet and savoury dishes. Couscous is very easy to make. I often steam some veges and garlic and just throw the couscous in near the end of cooking and let it sit. As I said before steamed vegetables and fish with salad and sliced avocado is one of the meals that makes me feel good afterwards.

Make your meals look good by adding some colour – cherry tomatoes, sliced avocado, parsley, sliced peppers

Learn about tofu and what brands you like. Readymade cans of organic cooked chickpeas and beans are an easy meal if you liven them up a bit.

These foods will provide a longer lasting energy and are less likely to be turned quickly into fat as white flour and sugar will be

The Short Cleansing Diet

Okay, I hate that word as much as you do, it just seems wrong and brings up bad memories and your Doctor probably won't recommend it. A cleansing diet is hard and not for everyone - but ..

If you have been eating a diet of white flour and processed food without much fibre for most of your life then there's a good chance your intestines and lower bowel are carrying sludge and layers of caked up gunk. I won't go into detail but autopsies have shown this. This gunk will prevent our bodies from obtaining the full benefit of the nutrients we eat

I'm not a fan of diets, they have a habit of coming back and biting you on the butt. You may lose weight but then it seems to sneak back on even worse than before. I wouldn't suggest a cleansing diet at all if we had all been eating a natural diet with plenty of vegetables and fruit. If you have you can probably skip this part. But a short cleansing diet will give your body a well needed rest, let your liver clean itself out and let that Important organ, the pancreas rest and get back to balance

Cleansing isn't for everyone. A gentle and slow introduction of more natural food to your diet over a long period of time is probably the best way. But for those of us who are Impatient and want instant results it could be worthwhile. Just don't expect that it will make handling your cravings any easier. If you are already badly our of balance it can make your cravings and mood swings temporarily worse

There are various ways you can do it. You can go for a full 10 day cleanse or just a brief 3 to 5 day one. Or if you are like me and have little willpower, just try it for a day or so.

I think my insides are already fairly clean. When I was in my twenty's I went on various fasts and did enemas and supplements. Once I ate only watermelons, pawpaw and coconut for an entire month.
Now I find it hard to fast even for a day unless I have a flu. But I'm not really a fan of fasting now. Water fasting used to be popular. It may be okay to do this if you are healthy and eat a high fibre diet, but for most of us you may feel very sick as your body begins to absorb all the toxins you have accumulated over the years!

So I suggest this cleansing diet to clean and purify yourself. You don't need to fast, just cut out all white flour and processed foods for as long as you can. You can eat - in fact I recommend it. But only light food such as salads, vegetables and fruit. If you're hungry eat some easy to digest, alkaline grains like buckwheat. High fibre food like this will act as a 'broom' sweeping your intestines, ridding you of waste and toxins.

This will work on a deep cellular level too. You need to make sure you drink enough water and herbal teas while you do this. At least 2 or 3 litres a day. I would also recommend using psyllium hulls or a detoxifying herbal supplements. These will contain specific herbs which will really help to clean out your lower bowels. The North American Indians took Cascara Sagrada, a sacred red tree bark whenever they were sick. I've taken it in capsule form

Normally I mix a teaspoon of Psyllium hulls in watered down juice and drink it. They taste a little bad but they are gentle on the body and help 'sweep out' your bowels being high in fibre.

If you are more adventurous you could take senna tablets. Psyllium and Senna are both available at your chemist. Psyllium is a seed husk and senna is also a seed but far more potent. I buy them in a pack for $16 and it says to take three or four. I'm a pro and take six, but a word of warning - make sure you are close to a toilet 8 to 10 hours later if you take Senna. The effects will be obvious and a little dramatic as you go rushing to the toilet with your butt cheeks squeezed together. And I guarantee you will be feeling quite 'cleansed' afterwards

I usually only take senna if I've been eating too much bread and cheese and I'm feeling a bit bunged up which is not a great feeling. Senna is a strong laxative, and eating more fibre rich vegetables, grains and fruit is a far more gentle and natural cleaner

What to expect during your cleanse:

The first day or two will usually be okay. It helps to get some books from the library on any type of fasting. They will inspire you as they go into sometimes shocking detail about how fasting will be cleansing the waste from your body. You should feel a little better, lighter. But there will be cravings. My advice is to use the emotional trigger change techniques and also to eat or drink something when you have a craving, but make it a healthy choice. Your favourite fruit or a nice salad. It's better to have something fibrous and healthy going through your body than a cream puff.

A small sacrifice you can make which won't adversely affect your cleanse is to add a small dollop of butter or olive oil and salt to some steamed vegetables, even a small amount of cheese. It's not ideal but its far better you stick to your plan and eat mainly veges than heating up a pizza! There will be plenty of time later - years in fact to eat all the pizza you want.

Some books will say that any eating will slow down your bodies natural healing processes. That's true to a point, but salads or fruit will assist the process and help clean out toxins from your bowels

The first day or three you will get hunger pangs. On about the third day something else happens. You will start to feel weak and get a headache. This is natural. For the first three to five days your body is absorbing and cleaning out all the junk and undigested food from your system. There are toxins in this and your body will be absorbing some of it into your bloodstream. This is why it's Important to keep eating fibre rich natural foods and Psyllium hulls as they will help your body to quickly clean out these toxins and lessen their reabsorption

But there is no avoiding the headache phase. It will usually only last for two or three days but you will feel lousy. Be gentle on yourself. Rest and drink lots of water. You may find yourself lying in bed for a lot of it, that's okay. But try to force yourself to do some gentle walking, stretching and breathing as this will help. Also do regular skin brushing. This is also a good time to take some additional vitamin C tablets or fresh lemon and honey drinks and antioxidants. Lemon is good here especially if you grind up the white pith and skin. These are rich in antioxidants and bioflavonoids but you will most likely need to mix it with honey. All red berries are rich in antioxidants

Antioxidants are natures little miracle cleaners and will attach themselves to toxins and random 'free radical' harmful cells, aiding your body in getting rid of them

If you go past day five you might get another surprise - you may start to worry as you don't feel hungry anymore! Don't worry as this is natural, your energy has been directed inward as your body is busy cleaning out years of accumulated waste and toxins from its intestines, bowels, organs and cells. Keep eating pure and cleansing foods and drink water or herbal tea regularly

The Cleansing diet may not work for everyone and if you have any sort of heart or medical condition talk to your doctor first. If you are a sugar addicted hypoglycaemic eating sweet fruit goes a bit against the goal of what we are trying to achieve here. But if eating it helps you stay on the cleanse go for it. But try to keep your fruit intake moderate. When I went on my hypoglycemic diet I would cycle to an orchard and buy fresh, unsprayed citrus to juice them. The book I was following said not to drink this but I'm sure it helped me. It felt pure and good

The Potassium Broth

This is an old trick from my fasting days. It works well with the cleansing diet and is easy to make. Our bodies are over acidic from eating processed foods and we need to make them more alkaline. Potassium does this. The broth includes potassium rich foods and the basic recipe is this:-
Simmer in a medium sized pot these ingredients:

Potatoes, and carrots - then add celery, garlic and dark leafy greens. Add a little sea salt. Iodised sea salt is best as the Iodine helps the cells rehydrate. Strain it and drink the broth, or if you are really hungry just eat the whole thing.
If you are being attacked by cravings and about to reach for the pizza, add a small amount of olive oil, butter or grated cheese. This broth is very satisfying and will help deacidify your body

Don't Eat Too Late At Night

A general rule of thumb is to eat simple meals in the morning, complex carbohydrate meals at midday and protein meals at night. Too much carbohydrate at night will be hard for your body to digest and most likely be turned to fat

Find Your Natural Appetite

Modern day foods have many additives and flavourings. This, combined with stuffing ourselves with hard to digest, processed and over refined white flour taxes our bodies and makes them work hard. We become locked in an addictive cycle of craving food which is harming us and doesn't provide hardly any nutrients.

Stuffed with all this cloggy white flour and processed food we quickly lose touch with our natural appetite and just want fat and sugar.

Our cravings are most likely because our body is craving vitamins and minerals. Eating lightly with fresh, alkaline food and exercise is the key here. Start to get used to that little pang of hunger. That's your natural appetite coming back. Instead of reaching for that sickeningly sweet snack bar and trading a few moments of euphoria for feeling tired and depressed, eat a handful of nuts or any slow release food to tide you over until you can have a decent meal with some fresh salad

A good way to keep cravings at bay is to take your liquorice twigs or tea to work. Take some nuts or healthy food with you. Any natural food will be better than a snack bar or cookies loaded with sugar

What To Drink?

I can't remember what I drank when I was young. I know there was a lot of milk and milo or hot chocolate, and probably a lot of juice and sachet drinks. I don't remember drinking water. All through until about 22 I remember drinking only fruit juice and fizzy drinks. I drank the cool and clean water of the mountains when I went climbing, but I hardly ever drank it otherwise. It just seemed tasteless

I tried many juice fasts when I was young, but drinking sweet fruit juice won't help a sugar addicted hypoglycaemic. We didn't have bottled water in shops back then. I didn't start to appreciate water until I went on a sugar free diet and got my taste buds back into balance

Water is good for you. You need to drink at least two litres a day. But drinking more between meals or in the morning is okay. Drinking a lot of water is one of the tricks bodybuilders use to shed weight. Drinking water will actually help your body to shed excess fluid. But Importantly, just remind yourself to drink enough

I often forget during the day. But now I have to take various pills sometimes so I always carry a water bottle with me. Clean water direct from a mountain stream or the rain is probably the best. Experiment with bottled brands as some are just cheap gimmicks from a tap and some will taste better than others.

I'm a fan of tea. I sometime have one good coffee a day in town but at home I drink a lot of black tea. I try to take other types of tea as well. Green Tea is extremely beneficial having properties which aid weight loss and benefit the liver. This is a great tea to have before you go to bed. Any of the fruit teas will be beneficial and will contain antioxidants. The liquorice tea is also a good one to have after a meal as it will help balance your blood sugar levels and stop those cravings for sweet things

You could get a good water filter for your kitchen sink and use this only for drinking. And if you have the money you could buy a water 'ioniser' or one of Dan Winters 'water spirals' This is new technology and it ranges from a double helix spiral that can be screwed onto a tap or a spiral encased in a box with magnets working on the water.

The spiral changes the structure water of the water making it softer or wetter. I won't go into technical detail, but this water is supposed to be more beneficial for you and may assist in hydrating and cleansing you at a deep cellular level

There is an Iranian Doctor by the name of Batmanghelidj who has been instructing Britains Head of Oncology at the Royal school of Medicine. Dr Batmanghelidj believes ALL illness is caused by dehydration, especially cancer and asthma. I've read some of his work and its very convincing though it is very technical and hard to understand. He has had great success at treating prison inmates who were suffering from various illnesses. Some had been tortured and starved. I remember he said that it can take a lot of time for our cells to properly rehydrate - months even. So carry that water bottle and don't forget to use it. It was Dr Batmanghelidj who said a small amount of sea salt and iodine was also needed with the water so our cells got the minerals they need

If you are addicted to sweet alcoholic drinks or fizzy drinks this can be a hard one. Living mostly sugar free will help. After a while you will find that these drinks taste overly sweet and you begin to wonder how you drank them before.
Kombucha can help. This is the Mongolian fungus which you grow in a large jar and add tea and honey or a little sugar. Kombucha is rich in enzymes and it will satisfy that craving you have for fizzy drinks or beer. One summer on Kombucha may be all you need to kick the habit. The Mongolians drank it before they went into battle

A soda stream could also be helpful. You can make your own healthy drinks from freshly squeezed citrus, peppermint tea or any natural flavour and add some honey. It's not ideal but it may help you kick the habit

Feeling Hungry

I can't lose weight for the life of me. When I was young I could fast for two weeks. Now I can't even go without food for one day. But I'm not into sudden radical changes anyway. I believe small dietary changes made over a long period of time are far more beneficial

Recently I got a really bad flu. At its peak I was laid up in bed for two days with tonsillitis. I couldn't talk and I was in great pain every time I swallowed. I spent $120 on various pain killing throat sprays, lozenges and organic cough syrup. A $4 pack of Aspirin proved to be the most effective relief

I sweated for 3 nights. The main part of the flu lasted a week but I felt the effects for a month. I couldn't eat anything except smoothies and I lost 12 kilos. I drank watered down fruit juice and finished with lemonade and ice cream sundaes. I lost weight but I turned my bloodstream into sugar and contracted diabetes

The one good thing about this event is that I got entirely used to the feeling of being a little hungry. My bloated stomach disappeared and I could feel that my stomach was pressing back into my spine - I felt skinny! What an odd feeling ... but I got used to it. A trigger event like this was the only way I could lose weight

The feeling of hunger wasn't too different from that churning pull you feel when you have a craving coming on, except that it was more controllable and it felt healthier. I actually felt a little high, kind of a warm and light feeling. It was helped by the hunger suppressing side effect of the diabetes pills I was taking, but the point I'm trying to make is that if you feel hungry, it's not the end of the world. Perhaps I'm stepping onto risky ground here as smaller, more regular meals are important for hypoglycaemics. But once we begin to heal and eat food with more nutrients, your body may not need to eat as much

Your overactive digestive organs have been continually pumping out their juices making you feel hungry. After a much needed rest they will begin to settle down and adjust to your new diet

I'm just asking you to acknowledge and recognise this feeling of true hunger, and when you feel it eat some protein or sustaining carbs to keep your blood sugar levels stable

Chapter Four

Other Helpful Information and Techniques

Skin Brushing and the Lymph System

The lymph system is very important. It's a network of vessels containing a clear lymph fluid comprising white blood cells and antibodies and its connected to our bloodstream.

Its job is to transport fluid upwards around the body, to carry out waste and rid the body of toxins with the antibodies that are produced in lymph nodes. There are 600 to 700 lymph nodes all around the body. You may have noticed if you have ever had an infection that you become sore under your arms or around your neck or groin? These are the lymph nodes working hard at producing antibodies. The tonsils are also lymph nodes

Swollen calves and feet in women (edema) is often a sign that your lymph system isn't working well. This is usually caused by being overweight, inactive or being stuck at a desk for a long time. The cure for this is good diet and exercise. If you walk or jog make sure you lie down and raise your legs afterwards, this will help to drain the lymph fluid which travels upwards through the body

Another technique which is beneficial to the lymphatic system is skin brushing. You need to find a natural bristle brush like a shoe brush. When you get out of bed, brush your entire body with it. You can feel the effect as it stimulates your circulation as well as shedding your body of old skin cells.

If you can find a bristle brush (I don't have one at the moment) you can try what I do, I'm using my hair brush. It's one with the little plastic bobbles on the ends. I find this massages my skin quite well, and then I use a loofah. That's one of those flat dried sea vegetables that you use in the bath. I haven't soaked mine but have kept it dry and it tends to cut and scrape the skin, but in a pleasurable way.

Take Notice of How You Feel After Eating

When you're addicted to food it all seems to happen so quickly and be a bit of a blur as you ride this roller coaster of emotions.

Try to slow things down a little. Take a few deep breaths before you eat to calm yourself. Say a word of thanks for the food you are about to eat. Try to start taking notice of how you feel after eating certain foods or food combinations – do you feel energised or tired? Is the food sitting like a rock and giving you a small stomach ache? Or is it giving you a warm glow inside your belly and making you feel light and energised?

These are valuable signs and worth taking note of. It may help to start keeping a small diary of which foods or meals gave you the best feeling? Because if you get a craving things can get out of control very quickly.

Wait a while after you eat. It can take 10 minutes for your body to absorb, register and react to what it is you've just eaten, so don't go rushing for the sweets or biscuits yet, give it a chance and the craving may disappear after a short while. Go and do a chore first

Do Diets Work?

For most of us? No. Because we are addicts and we use food like a drug. This leads to a situation of swings and roundabouts where any short term weight loss you have shed will inexorably be put back on over time. You could possibly end up being heavier!

How these people in the ads have managed to turn from a whale into a normal sized person I don't know. They obviously aren't hypoglycaemic and they must have incredible willpower.

Diets don't work for me. A 'Life Change' of eating well does. By bringing in healthy foods into my daily life and cutting out all the processed junk. And by remaining active and getting back in touch with my natural appetite

Smoothie's

Smoothie's can be helpful. The problem with them if you are hypoglycemic is that they are based on either fruit juice or some type of milk which can upset your balance. As I said when I talked about my flu and couldn't eat, I drank smoothies and ended up getting diabetes.

Use rice, almond or oat milk in moderation. If you are hypoglycaemic it's probably best to stay away from smoothies for now, unless you can construct one with just water, banana, avocado etc. Or perhaps a blended seed / nut drink with carob and cold pressed flax seed oil

Weight Loss Programs

Any help we can get to lose weight is probably a good thing and the structure of recognised weight loss programs can be helpful. I went on a very common one. It was slightly unusual in that it used everyday food and didn't put an emphasis on eating more vegetables. But that can be okay for a start

What it did show me was the food value of many of our common foods. I was surprised to learn that one piece of battered fish was one third of my entire daily food intake, as was 2 scoops of ice cream, one matchbox sized block of cheese or two rows of chocolate from a king size bar. For many women of shorter stature these foods can make up almost half of your daily intake

This was really helpful. If you had a choice between a small cube of cheese or a full bowl of stir fry with colourful vegetables and some meat or tofu – which one would you choose to eat as a meal?

I did manage to gradually lose weight and stick to it so it was working for me. You may have noticed that I don't talk about weight loss in this book. If you eat healthily, remain active and especially cut out starchy and junk food, the weight will drop off naturally and quickly.

Do Things That Make You Feel Good

During this healing phase and dietary change be gentle on yourself.
Don't be too hard on yourself if you 'break the rules'. Be forgiving as you have all your life left and plenty of time left to get it right, just don't give up – the rewards of better mobility, better mood and health WILL be worth it.

Treat yourself to other things you enjoy that don't involve eating. Although eating a good vegetarian meal at a restaurant can be a good reward too.

Depression

Sometimes others don't understand depression. A friend of mine once looked down her nose at me when I described mine and said "I can't understand that, if I feel depressed I just do something about it". She was a Leo and a very capable and confident woman. I told her that it's like being on a ladder and we are all on different rungs. And that if you slip down far enough the world seems like a very black place and you can't get out of the feeling that easily

Six years later she walked right up to me and said "I know what you mean". And she described how she had tried to get into journalism school but had been rejected

If you feel depression coming on do something to snap out of it. You know what's going to happen if you let yourself become depressed – you will spiral down to that dark place and feel sorry for yourself for a week or more.

As hard as it is, try and force yourself to break this cycle. Exercise helps, a walk on the beach or in the mountains. Go and get a massage and be pampered. Whatever you need to do to feel good about yourself. We often sacrifice our lives a lot for others and forget to take some time out for ourselves. Do it, you deserve it

I got some help from a book by Osho or Bhagwan Shree Rajneesh. He said that all emotions are transient and they only hang around if we negate them. That's exactly what I was doing – waking up everyday, feeling depressed and thinking that I was a failure because my school friends all had good jobs and weren't depressed.

He says to just go with the feeling and don't negate it. Explore it – there are even some beautiful sides to depression. And after this if I woke up depressed I would just think ..."hah, that's interesting" and get on with my day. I did have the luxury of lots of spare time where I sat down and wrote about the reasons why I was depressed. I then worked on them one by one. This involved going on an outdoor course and a music workshop, both of which boosted my self-esteem a lot

Sex, Marijuana and Alcohol

These are best avoided during this healing phase. They are all intense things which have the risk of throwing you a little out of balance, and all three of them will usually give you an appetite. I personally find that drinking one small bottle of beer will make me hungry when I wasn't hungry before

You Will Always Be An Alcoholic

I think this is one of the basic premises of Alcoholics Anonymous, that even when you kick your addiction you will always be an alcoholic and you need to be ever vigilant.

It's very much the same with hypoglycemia. I managed to kick mine completely and then for a year after that I could eat the occasional sweet biscuit and actually stop after one or two. This would have been Impossible for me before. The warning signs are when you start getting cravings again. I can easily slip back into being unhealthy if I don't remain vigilant all the time. My tendency is that when I begin to feel good I will become over confident and start eating sweet foods again.

But even when you think you are healed it actually takes quite a few months for your body to fully adjust to these changes and stabilise itself

What will happen to me if I don't do anything?

Any physical ailments you have now will most likely only get worse over time if you don't stop this cycle. Your overworked organs will work even more poorly and this will put strain on your entire body. Your digestive organs can enlarge to two or three times their size and you may have problems with inflammation affecting your mobility and quality of life

I got psoriatic arthritis. All of a sudden I found I couldn't walk properly in the morning - the balls of my feet were sore and I limped around until 1pm when I warmed up a bit. I went and saw various doctors but it was six years until I was diagnosed.

One sign of psoriatic arthritis is that you may get a flaky scalp or red sores on your scalp, or a swollen large toe or thumb. Another symptom can be muscle aches that make it hard to walk or get out of your chair. Psoriatic arthritis is nothing to do with your joints, mine are perfectly healthy. It's your own Immune system attacking itself

My muscles got sore and if I bruised or sprained any area of my body it would inflame and be sore for months afterwards. If I slip on my diet now I will get this very quickly, my hands and feet begin to ache and I can barely get out of bed and walk to the kitchen. I occasionally have to take 800 mg of Brufen or strong ibuprofen. At my worst I was taking 3 of these a day for 4 years

If the liver is toxic and struggling to do its job many people get headaches and migraines.

For me, I've found the best solution is a good diet with lots of vegetables, regular exercise, drinking plenty of water and herb teas and eating lightly – especially in the evening. If I overeat at night with too much carbohydrate or sugar I will get sore straight away

Diabetes will also be waiting in the wings for you if you don't heal hypoglycemia. My markers were good until I was about 48 and I got diabetes when I was 51.

Afterword

You may have noticed a few oxymoronic statements in this book where I'm recommending foods or food combinations which I've said are unhealthy. That's because if you're a full on food addict you will need some 'backstops' – things to eat which may not be ideal but are still more on the healthy side and will be a far better option than eating an entire packet of chocolate biscuits

If you're a full on food addict you need to be forgiving with yourself and you may need to wean yourself gradually off your addictive foods. I'm not saying you can't eat KFC or McDonalds ever again. Make these foods more of a treat for special occasions. And when you eat them have some coleslaw and don't have the cheap fizzy drink

If any of you are having suicidal thoughts I really feel for you. I know what it's like, and it's a rare person who can empathise and understand it unless they've actually been there

My advice is don't do it. Suicide doesn't rid us of our problems. We will only have to come and deal with them in our next life. And suicide is selfish in a way, because so many other people are adversely affected and suffer because of it – think of the person in your family who you love the most - and think about how much they will suffer if you leave so suddenly. Stay here for their sake.

But I do want you all to selfishly look after yourselves and do the things you need to do to get back to health. Because only then can we start to do the real work in life - helping others. It's the only thing I've found that gives me deep joy and happiness, everything else is just temporary

I wish you all the best on your journey. It may not be an easy one. I feel I was lucky to have survived mine, so I hope this short book will help some of you to survive yours.

Love, peace, health and serenity to you all

Tony